CDC
State Heart Disease and Stroke Prevention Program

Evaluation Framework

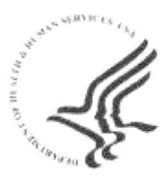

DEPARTMENT OF HEALTH AND HUMAN SERVICES
CENTERS FOR DISEASE CONTROL AND PREVENTION
NATIONAL CENTER FOR CHRONIC DISEASE PREVENTION
AND HEALTH PROMOTION

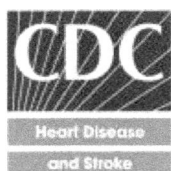

Acknowledgements

This document was developed by the Centers for Disease Control and Prevention (CDC), National Center for Chronic Disease Prevention and Health Promotion, Division of Adult and Community Health, State Heart Disease and Stroke Prevention programs. Sheree Marshall Williams, Ph.D., was the lead author and was assisted by ORC Macro and members of the Cardiovascular Health Branch's team for Program Services, Intervention, and Evaluation (PSIE). The logic model was developed by the PSIE with assistance from ORC Macro and Thomas Chapel and Bobby Milstein of CDC. The *Evaluation Framework for the State Heart Disease and Stroke Prevention Programs* and the logic model were further refined through helpful suggestions from the programs' managers and the evaluation coordinators in states receiving comprehensive funding from CDC's Heart Disease and Stroke Prevention Program. For more information about the logic model and evaluation framework, contact the Cardiovascular Health Branch at CDC at 770–488–2424.

1. Introduction

Among men and women, and across all racial and ethnic groups, heart disease and stroke are among our nation's leading killers and leading causes of disability. Although most of the major risk factors for heart disease and stroke are modifiable or preventable, over 80 percent of Americans report having at least one major risk factor or related condition. These include high blood pressure, high blood cholesterol, tobacco use, physical inactivity, poor diet, obesity, and diabetes. In addition, major disparities exist among population groups, with certain racial/ethnic groups and other priority populations having substantially higher rates of death and disability from cardiovascular diseases than the overall population.

Recognizing the immense burden of cardiovascular disease (CVD), Congress made funding available in FY 1998 to initiate a national, state-based CVD prevention program. The State Heart Disease and Stroke Prevention Program is administered by the Centers for Disease Control and Prevention (CDC). Through categorical funding, the State Heart Disease and Stroke Prevention Program is designed to increase the leadership of state health departments in cardiovascular health promotion and cardiovascular disease prevention and control and to expand and direct efforts to establish a national CVH program.

As states conduct activities related to CVH promotion and CVD prevention, they will want to evaluate their programs. The purpose of this evaluation framework is to help states and partners understand CDC's goals for CVH State Program evaluation and the importance of using evaluation information for planning and program improvement. This document outlines suggested program activities and evaluation goals for participating states.

II. CDC's Framework for Program Evaluation

Program evaluation is a systematic way of measuring the success of public health programs. The Heart Disease and Stroke Prevention Program's evaluation framework is based on CDC's evaluation framework, a practical tool designed to summarize and organize the essential elements of any program evaluation. This framework consists of six steps, which are depicted in Figure 1 and described briefly below. More information regarding CDC's evaluation framework can be found on the internet at http://www.cdc.gov/mmwr/PDF/RR/RR4811.pdf or in the CDC document *"Framework for Program Evaluation in Public Health"* (CDC, 1999) .

FIGURE 1. Recommended framework for program evaluation

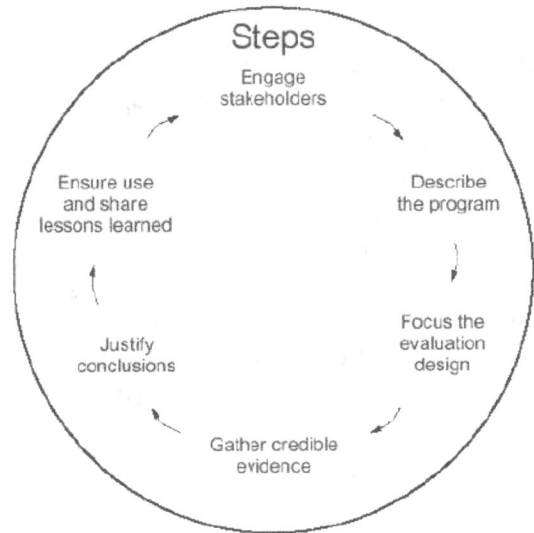

1. **Engage stakeholders**
   - Engage those who might have an interest or stake in the issues addressed by the program from the beginning stages of the program.

2. **Describe the Program**
   - This description should convey the mission and objectives of the program and set the frame of reference for evaluation decisions.

3. **Focus the evaluation design**
   - Identify issues of greatest concern to stakeholders, the questions to be asked in the evaluation, and the methods used to develop the questions.

4. **Gather credible evidence**
   - The more credible the evidence is, the more credible will be the evaluation findings and the recommendations that follow from them.

5. **Justify conclusions**
   - Evaluation conclusions should be based on the evidence gathered, and program's success should be judged against agreed-upon

values or standards set by the stakeholders prior to conducting the evaluation.

6. **Ensure that lessons learned are shared and applied**.
   - Program participants should make a deliberate effort to disseminate the evaluation processes they use and the findings of their evaluations so that other entities conducting CVH projects can learn from their experience.

2. Heart Disease and Stroke Prevention Program Description

Goals of CDC's Heart Disease and Stroke Prevention Program

- Increase the **capacity** of states to promote CVH and prevent and control CVD.
- Conduct **surveillance** of CVD, CVD-related risk factors, and policy and environmental sectors that support CVH.
- Develop, implement, and improve **program interventions** to promote CVH and prevent and control CVD.
- Identify intervention **"models that work"** in promoting CVH and preventing and controlling CVD.
- **Eliminate disparities** in CVH between general and priority populations.

The Heart Disease and Stoke Prevention Program goals involve changing environmental and policy systems that affect people's cardiovascular health as well as increasing education, training, assessment, and communication to prevent and control CVD. To meet these goals, programs attempt to influence those in a position to make policy changes to improve the cardiovascular health of individuals (e.g., health care providers, school principals, business managers). To be effective, an intervention plan should use educational, policy, and environmental strategies.

Environmental change interventions are used to change both the physical and social environment to influence people's attitudes and health behaviors. One way to produce environmental change is through policy changes that can be divided into changes in legislative/regulatory policies and changes in organizational policies. **Legislative/regulatory policies** are formal policies that have been written into laws and affect the general public. **Organizational policies** are those that specific organizations, such as schools, businesses, or health care providers, create to define appropriate behavior within the confines of their organization. These policies may not affect the general public, but they do affect those who frequent the locations where the policies are in place (Schmid et al., 1995).

To accomplish their goals, state heart disease and stroke prevention Programs should engage in capacity building, surveillance, and program interventions. Capacity building and program interventions both contribute directly to targeted policy changes, while **surveillance** activities are used to help to target areas where policy changes should occur. These three components are complementary, and each is necessary if a state heart disease and stroke prevention program is to be effective. Each of these components is discussed in greater depth below, and a glossary of terms related to the heart disease and stroke prevention program is included in Appendix A.

Capacity building. Capacity building refers to efforts by state health departments to build the assets, resources, and commitments necessary to improve their residents' cardiovascular health by supporting population-based interventions that emphasize policy and environmental changes at the system level.

The following eight activities are intended to help states build the capacity of their health department:

1. ***Develop and coordinate partnerships.*** States should develop new partnerships and enhance existing partnerships with (1) traditional partners within and outside the state health department, (2) nontraditional organizations (e.g., transportation, urban planning, parks and recreation, health care organizations), and (3) organizations that address a CVD risk factor or serve priority populations. By involving these organizations to promote cardiovascular health, states will help increase coordination among partners and avoid duplicating cardiovascular disease prevention efforts.

2. ***Develop the scientific capacity to define the cardiovascular disease burden and to evaluate programs.*** By enhancing their capacity in epidemiology, behavioral science, statistics, surveillance, and data analysis, states can better analyze existing data such as vital statistics, hospital discharge data, and Behavioral Risk Factor Surveillance System (BRFSS) data. These data sources are used to track trends and identify patterns or disparities in the CVD burden by geography, gender, race, ethnicity, and socioeconomic status.

3. ***Develop an inventory of policies and environmental sectors that promote CVH***. States should assess existing policies and environments that support positive CVH behaviors at

the state level, as well as in communities, schools, worksites, and health care facilities.

4. ***Develop or update a state CVH plan***. States should work with partners to develop a comprehensive state plan with population-based objectives and strategies to promote CVH and reduce the prevalence of CVD and related risk factors.

5. ***Provide training and technical assistance***. States should provide training to help state and local health department staff, partners, and other organizations better promote CVH.

6. ***Develop population-based strategies***. States should identify population-based strategies to promote CVH as well as promote the prevention and control of CVD and related risk factors.

7. ***Develop culturally competent strategies for addressing priority populations.*** States should identify intervention strategies specific to priority populations.

8. ***Develop a CVH infrastructure within the state health department.*** States should develop program and managerial infrastructure to support CVH activities by hiring program, evaluation, and epidemiologic staff and identifying additional resources.

Surveillance. CVD epidemiologic data are compiled from data in existing surveillance systems such as state BRFSS surveys and mortality and morbidity reports. These surveillance systems track changes in rates of CVD and related risk factors. States should use surveillance information to increase their scientific or epidemiologic capacity to define the CVD burden, (see item 2 of capacity building). States should also use surveillance data when setting priorities for program planning, developing a state CVH plan, identifying priorities for policy and environmental interventions, improving evaluation capacity, and identifying priority populations.

Program Interventions. Program interventions should focus on policy and environmental strategies as well as on educating people about CVH. Interventions are implemented at both the state level and in communities, schools, worksites, and health care facilities.

IV. Logic Model for the State Heart Disease and Stroke Prevention Programs

Logic models are commonly used to graphically depict the organization, structure, assumptions, and associations underlying a program. Some logic models are fully descriptive and include all aspects of program structure, organization, and expected outcomes in addition to a theoretical framework. For instance, the logic model for the State Heart Disease and Stroke Prevention Program is based on a socioecological model, which links environmental and policy systems changes with individual-level behavioral changes (McLeroy et al., 1988). This logic model depicts relationships and actions that are expected to precede long-term changes in CVD rates.

It is important to note that logic models are often cyclical rather than linear in that information obtained during a particular activity can be used to modify another activity even if that activity precedes it in the logic model. For example, a state plan for CVH activities influences the development of a work plan for implementing CVH activities and the work plan can impact portions of the state plan. Similarly developing the state plan can affect capacity- building activities. Thus the CVH logic model is dynamic with any number of activities providing input into different aspects of the model. The feedback loops in the model are the strongest anticipated influences but do not exhaust all the possible influences.

Logic models not only serve to describe the program, but they also act as a tool to guide program evaluation. By identifying the steps necessary to reach intended outcomes, the logic model helps users determine the program evaluation focus.

Two logic models have been developed to describe the CVH State Program and its intended effects. The overview logic model provides a general overview of the program, and the expanded logic model provides a more detailed description. These logic models primarily depict the activities and effects intended *by CDC funding* to states; however, because CDC may be only one of several funding sources, the logic model for a particular state's overall CVH efforts may be more elaborate than these models. The logic models provide an explanation of how capacity building, surveillance, and intervention activities are affected by CDC and state activities.

The **overview logic model**, shown in Appendix B, depicts the major activities and intended outcomes of the program. The activities of capacity

9

building, surveillance, and interventions lead to improved health status through a series of changes in policies and environments and individual behavior. "System changes" are defined as those modifications in policy and environments that take place at the state and community level that affect the population targeted. Once policies and environmental systems and infrastructure to support heart-healthy lifestyles are in place, individual behavioral change is more likely to occur. As a result of these individual behavioral changes, the health status of the targeted population is expected to improve, leading to a decrease in death and disability rates and eliminating CVD disparities between the general and priority populations.

An **expanded logic model** was developed to elaborate the processes and events that occur between the time state activities are implemented and the time changes in long-term health outcomes can be detected. (See Appendix C.) This model outlines CDC and state activities in terms of capacity building, surveillance, and interventions. Both the CDC and state activities are designed to produce short-term outcomes such as the development of a work plan and strategies for system level changes, the effective implementation of interventions, and actions by target audiences and change agents (those who are in the position to influence others). These outcomes are designed to change policies and environmental factors that lead to behavioral changes and improved health among members of the target population and ultimately to a decrease death and disability rates and eliminate CVD disparities between general and priority populations. For a more detailed explanation of each of the logic models, see Appendix D.

IV. State Grantee Levels

CDC funds state programs at Capacity Building and Basic Implementation support levels. Although the expectations for states funded at these different levels overlap, they are somewhat different.

A. Capacity Building Programs

States funded at the capacity-building level build capacity through the eight activities described below.

1. Develop and coordinate partnerships.
2. Develop the scientific capacity to define the cardiovascular disease burden within the state and to evaluate programs.
3. Develop an inventory of policy and environmental supports.
4. Develop or update a state CVH plan.
5. Provide training and technical assistance.
6. Develop population-based strategies.
7. Develop culturally competent strategies for priority populations.
8. Develop a CVH infrastructure within the state health department.

Capacity-building states build a core capacity that allow them to implement effective interventions. These capacity-building activities are indicated under the "process" heading and the first two columns under "short-term outcomes" in the expanded logic model.

B. Basic Implementation Programs

States funded at the basic-implementation level conduct the following activities:

1. Continue, strengthen, and enhance the eight core state activities.
2. Implement, disseminate, and evaluate intervention activities throughout the state, including those of state-level organizations and those at specified settings (communities, worksites, schools, health care facilities).
3. Implement strategies for addressing priority populations.
4. Monitor secondary prevention strategies (e.g., hypertension and cholesterol control, aspirin and drug therapy, hormone replacement therapy, dietary changes) by monitoring data collected by peer reviewed organizations (PRO), and other appropriate groups.

5. Implement professional education activities for health care providers and change agents (e.g., politicians, school principals) to promote the use of appropriate primary and secondary prevention practices and standards of care.

The goal of basic implementation states is to implement and/or influence policy and environmental changes (the intermediate outcome in the expanded logic model) that promote CVH and reduce rates of CVD.

The vision underlying the State Heart Disease and Stroke Prevention Program is that all states will become Basic Implementation states and conduct CVH interventions. As their CVH capacity and infrastructure increase and as resources become available, Capacity Building states can apply to become Basic Implementation states. It should be noted that although CDC's expectations for Capacity Building and Basic Implementation states differ, the activities of states occur along a continuum as shown in the expanded logic model. However, there is no standard for how long a state should or will take to move from "Capacity Building" to "Basic Implementation" status.

VI. Program Evaluation

An important component of any program is the evaluation of its effectiveness from the earliest stages of implementation. Program evaluation is a systematic way to account for public health actions and to provide data for program improvement. The purpose of CVH State Program evaluation is to document that participating state programs are achieving their goals and progressing toward their intended long-term outcomes.

**Evaluation Goals for CDC's Heart Disease
And Stroke Prevention Program**

- Document changes in state **capacity** to address CVH.
- Systematically document CVD burden using **surveillance** data.
- Document changes in CVH **policies and environmental factors that support CVH.**
- Document the process of implementing interventions and the impact of **interventions** at the state and local level, in particular settings, and in priority populations.

Evaluation methodology for the State Heart Disease and Stroke Prevention Program involves separate evaluations of *capacity building, surveillance, and policy and environmental interventions*. Evaluation does not have to include comparison communities or quasi-experimental designs but should rely upon existing data systems for comparison data. States are encouraged to use process evaluation methods to (1) evaluate how policy and environmental strategies were implemented, (2) evaluate the extent to which their program is being implemented as intended, and (3) determine whether their program is appropriately focusing its CVH efforts, especially toward priority populations.

A. Capacity Building

Purpose
To determine whether state health departments have increased their capacity to perform tasks needed to address heart disease and stroke in a

comprehensive manner and to reach the long-term goals of the Cardiovascular Health State Program.

Evaluation Question(s)
What progress has been made in addressing the eight components of capacity building?

Expectations for Capacity Building and Basic Implementation States
Demonstrate an increasing ability over time to perform the eight core capacity-building activities, as measured by the semi-annual report.

Data Collection
CDC's CVH Branch has developed a suggested semiannual reporting form (available upon request) that states can use to track their capacity building. The reporting form includes information on the eight capacity-building activities discussed in the program description.

B. Surveillance

Purpose
1. To collect epidemiologic data from the BRFSS, mortality and morbidity reports, hospital discharge data, and other state-based data sources so changes in a population's CVD burden and related risk factors and conditions can be tracked.
2. To aggregate years of BRFSS data for priority populations to determine whether CVD rates have changed or if CVD disparities have been reduced.
3. To collect data on existing policies and environmental changes across states using established indicators.
4. To monitor use of secondary prevention strategies (through Peer Reviewed Organizations data and other appropriate data sources).

Evaluation Questions
1. What changes are occurring in the state population's CVD burden and risk factors over time?
2. What changes are occurring specifically in priority populations over time?
3. What policy and environmental changes have taken place over time?
4. What changes are occurring in the use of secondary prevention strategies over time?

Expectations for Capacity Building

1. Demonstrate the scientific capacity to define the cardiovascular disease burden for their state.
2. Demonstrate the ability to track the following **trends** in CVD in the general population and priority populations over time: CVD mortality, morbidity, disability, and risk factors; patients' age at onset of CVD, and the disparity in these factors between general and priority populations. States should collect cardiovascular-related data using the protocols and time line. We recommend that states collect data using the BRFSS modules on hypertension awareness, cholesterol awareness, and cardiovascular disease. We also recommend that funded states collect data using the BRFSS Module on heart attack and stroke signs and symptoms at least every four years or, if possible, every two years.
3. Publish a document describing the state CVD burden every 5 years and collect burden data at least every 2 years or as needed for program planning.

Expectations for Basic Implementation States

Basic Implementation states should meet the three expectations for core states plus the following:

1. Demonstrate that they have collected and analyzed indicators of CVH-related policies and environmental supports for CVH.
2. Demonstrate that they can collect data on secondary prevention strategies at least every two years or as needed for program planning.

Data Collection

The following are the main variables to consider when measuring a populations' CVD burden:

- Race/ethnicity
- Age
- Gender
- Socioeconomic status (SES)
- Deaths due to heart disease and stroke
- CVD prevalence and average age of CVD patients at disease onset
- CVD disability rates
- Prevalence of CVD risk factors:
  - High blood pressure
  - High blood cholesterol
  - Tobacco use

- Poor nutrition
- Physical inactivity
- CVD-related conditions:
- Obesity
- Diabetes
- Knowledge of signs and symptoms
- Secondary Prevention

C. Program Intervention

Purpose
To monitor the implementation and outcomes of the program interventions.

Evaluation Questions
- Did CVH program interventions influence policy or environmental supports?
- Did educational interventions increase public awareness of CVD (e.g., its signs and symptoms)?
- Were interventions implemented as expected?
- Were program evaluation results used for program improvement and to identify "models that work"?
- Were interventions conducted in priority populations using culturally appropriate strategies?

Expectations for Capacity Building States
Capacity Building states are not expected to implement major population-based interventions. If Capacity Building states choose to conduct pilot interventions or receive supplemental funds for interventions, the interventions should be evaluated.

Expectations for Basic Implementation States
1. Develop and implement population-based intervention strategies for general and priority populations.
2. Show that interventions result in policy and environmental changes. Educational interventions should increase public awareness of CVH and CVD issues, increase support for policy and environmental changes to improve people's CVH, and increase public knowledge about the signs and symptoms of CVD. Over time, states should address policy and environmental changes at the state level, in all four settings, in the general population, and in all priority populations. In addition, they should document anticipated and unanticipated outcomes, lessons

16

learned, and "models that work" and use these findings for program improvement.

Data Collection

Basic Implementation states should provide process and outcome data and other information regarding setting- and state-level interventions. Information to be provided includes the following:

- A brief description of the intervention
- Program objective(s)
- Documentation of whether the objective was met
- Demographic characteristics of the population served by the intervention
- Setting(s) for the intervention (i.e., community, school, worksite, health care facility)
- The geographic region in which the intervention was conducted
- Materials developed
- The target disease (e.g., heart disease, stoke)
- Risk factors addressed (e.g., hypertension, high cholesterol, tobacco use, obesity, nutrition)
- Healthy People 2010 objectives addressed
- Policy changes achieved
- Environmental changes achieved
- Outcome measures to be used
- Lessons learned
- The intervention's impact on participants
- The intervention's impact on the setting
- The theoretical model used for the intervention

Table 1
Summary of CVH Program Components and Related Activities

Program Component	Activities
State Capacity Building	• Develop the scientific capacity to define the cardiovascular disease burden and to evaluate programs. • Develop an inventory of policies and environmental supports. • Develop or update a state CVH plan. • Provide training and technical assistance. • Develop population-based strategies. • Develop culturally competent strategies for priority populations. • Develop a CVH infrastructure within the state health department

Surveillance	• Behavioral Risk Factor Surveillance Survey (BRFSS)
	  CVD Module
	  Hypertension
	  Cholesterol
	  Heart Attack and Stroke Signs and Symptoms
	  Tobacco
	  Nutrition
	  Physical Activity
	  Obesity
	  Diabetes
	• Peer review organization (PRO) data
	• Policy and environmental indicators
	• Mortality data
	• Hospital discharge data

Program Intervention+	• State-level and local-level interventions • Setting-level interventions • Interventions in different contexts including priority population interventions, and culturally appropriate interventions

+ Evaluation results from selected CVH interventions will be reviewed and summarized.

References

Cited References

Centers for Disease Control and Prevention. Framework for program evaluation in public health. *Morbidity and Mortality Weekly Report* 1999;48(RR11):1-40.

McLeroy K, Bibeau D, Steckler A, Glanz K. An ecological perspective on health promotion programs. *Health Education Quarterly* 1998;15:351-377.

Schmid TL, Pratt M, Howze E. Policy as intervention: environmental and policy approaches to the prevention of cardiovascular disease. *American Journal of Public Health* 1985;85:1207
-12ll.

Additional References

Brownson RC, Matson-Koffman D, Novotny T.E, Huges RG, Eriksen MR. Environmental and policy interventions to control tobacco use and prevent cardiovascular disease. *Health Education Quarterly* 1995;22:478-498.

Glanz K, Lankenau B, Foerster S, Temple S, Mullis R, Schmid T. Environmental and policy approaches to cardiovascular disease prevention through nutrition: opportunities for state and local action. *Health Education Quarterly* 1995;22:512-527.

Jeffery RW, French SA. Environmental influences on eating and physical activity. *American Journal of Public Health* 1998;88:277-280.

King AC, Jeffery RW, Fridinger F, Dusenbury L, Provence S, Hedlund SA, Spangler K. Environmental and policy approaches to cardiovascular disease prevention through physical activity: Issues and opportunities. *Health Education Quarterly* 1995;22:499-527.

Nestle M, Jacobson MF. Halting the obesity epidemic: A public health policy approach. *Public Health Reports* 2000;115:12-24.

Sallis JF, Bauman A, Pratt M. Environmental and policy interventions to promote physical activity. *American Journal of Preventive Medicine* 1998;15:379-397.

W.K. Kellogg Foundation. Using logic models to bring together planning, evaluation, and action: *Logic Model Development Guide 2000*. Item #1209. Available at http:www.wkkf.org. (Accessed June 2004.)

Cardiovascular Health (CVH) Plan: A written document specifying current state-level goals, objectives, and activities for cardiovascular health promotion and disease prevention and control. Strategies should emphasize policy and environmental approaches to improving CVH as well as education to increase support for policy and environmental changes. The plan should be comprehensive, with population-based interventions. Activities should be coordinated among state's partners.

Champion: A person (either within or outside of the state health department) who advocates for legislation, policy changes, resources, or state funding to support the CVH State Program. A champion has leadership skills, special status, or abilities to leverage resources or convince others of the importance of this program and its activities.

Capacity: For the CDC's Heart Disease and Stroke Prevention Program, capacity is defined as the assets, resources, and commitment necessary to improve a population's cardiovascular health by supporting population-based interventions that emphasize policy and environmental strategies. Capacity has been operationally defined as the seven components required of grantees, in addition to their CVH infrastructure.

Change agent: A person who has the ability to make changes in policies and environments. For example, a change agent in a school might be the principal and at a work site might be the manager.

Community: A social unit that usually encompasses a geographic region in which residents live and interact socially, such as a political subunit (e.g., a county or town) or a smaller area (e.g., a neighborhood or a housing complex). A community may also be a social organization (a formal or informal group of people who share common interests, such as a faith organization). In reality, an individual may be a member of several communities or subgroups defined by a variety of factors, such as age, sex, occupation, socioeconomic status, activities, culture, or history.

Basic Implementation Program: A funding level for the CDC Cardiovascular State Program that allows states to continue and enhance core capacity functions. States with basic implementation funding are expected to implement, disseminate, and evaluate intervention activities throughout and within the state, within state-level organizations, and at various settings; monitor secondary prevention strategies; complement professional education activities; and extend resources to local health agencies, communities, and organizations. Both CDC-funded Basic Implementation and Core Capacity program activities would be a part of an overall state CVH plan, although there may be strategies, objectives, and activities in the plan other than those funded by CDC.

Contact: For the purposes of evaluation reporting, a "contact" is establishing communication with a person or organization for enhancing cardiovascular health among populations to support the state cardiovascular program.

Core Capacity-funded Programs: A funding level for the CDC Cardiovascular State Program that allows sates to build capacity, commitment, and resources to develop basic CVD health promotion, disease prevention, and control functions and activities. They are asked to do this by (1) developing partnerships and coordinating program related to primary and secondary prevention, (2) developing the scientific capacity to define the CVD burden, (3) developing an inventory of policies and environments that support positive CVH behaviors, (4) developing a state plan for CVH promotion, (5) providing training and technical assistance, (6) developing population-based intervention strategies, (7) developing culturally competent strategies for addressing priority populations, and (8) developing a CVH infrastructive within the state health department.

Culturally competent Interventions: Interventions that have been designed with guidance from relevant cultural or population groups and that demonstrate sensitivity to the cultural dimensions of risk factors and behaviors important for cardiovascular health.

Environment: A community encompassing all settings for which policies, social, and physical space can be manipulated at some level. Examples include retail businesses (e.g., restaurants, grocers) and public space such as parks, sidewalks, and green ways. Environmental changes would, therefore, be those changes necessary to foster and maintain individual-level behavioral changes to improve cardiovascular health.

Environmental change interventions: Interventions designed to influence people's attitudes and health behaviors by changing or altering both the physical and social environment.

Evaluation: A process of measuring components critical to the success of a state cardiovascular health program, including surveillance, program monitoring, and formative evaluation. Evaluation should address strategy implementation, changes in policies and the physical and social environments affecting cardiovascular health, and, ultimately, changes in behavioral risk factors.

Focus areas: The areas identified for attention by the CVH State Program, including physical activity, nutrition, secondary prevention, and control of hypertension and hypercholesterolemia.

Indicators: Factors that provide a measure or index of cardiovascular health similar to the way "economic indicators" measure economic health. In the Cardiovascular Health State Program, the indicators measure policies and environmental factors associated with reduced rates of (CVD and CVD risk factors and related conditions (tobacco use, hypertension, high cholesterol, physical inactivity, and poor nutrition). Indicators include restaurants with smoke-free policies, schools with policies that require daily physical education, worksites with cafeterias and vending machines that offer heart-healthy food and beverage choices, and health care organizations that adopt quality standards of care for primary and secondary prevention of CVD. Indicators are a way to obtain information about the intermediate effects of a health promotion effort that will in turn lead to individual behavioral changes, improve people's health status, and reduce CVD rates.

Intervention: The part of a strategy, incorporating method and technique, that actually reached a person or population.

Inventory: A written assessment of existing policies and environmental conditions that either promote or impede, cardiovascular health in a specified setting at the state, regional, or community level. States must justify the geographical subunit selected in their work plan and ensure that it is appropriate for assisting them with their CVH plan. The process of conducting an inventory must be systematic and rational with face validity, but the data collection procedure need not necessarily be randomized nor must the scale be validated.

The information in an inventory is used to determine the policy and environmental interventions and activities to be addressed and evaluated by the state CVH program. For example, if the inventory shows that the state has policies requiring schools to be tobacco-free, then the program might not focus on this policy issue when working in the school setting.

An inventory should focus on one or more of the following areas: physical activity, nutrition, and secondary prevention of CVD, including reducing elevated blood pressure or an elevated cholesterol level. For example, an inventory for nutrition in the school setting could include food service policies, the existence of vending machines and their contents, and student access to fast food sites near school; an inventory for physical activity in the community setting could include the availability of sidewalks, access to walking trails and parks, and zoning policies requiring green space and bike lanes; and an inventory for secondary prevention in health care settings could include standards of care for those with cardiovascular disease or hypertension, follow-up practices used to promote compliance with medication, and insurance coverage for treating cardiovascular disease.

An inventory should be conducted when a state first enters the CVH State Program and during project years 02 to 05; additional inventories should be conducted in at least one of each of the four settings (i.e., communities, health care sites, worksites, and schools). As CVH State Program inventory tools are developed or identified by individual states, Prevention Research Centers, and CDC, the tools will be made available for use by other states.

Partnerships:
A. **Partnerships within the state health department:**. Because organizational structures vary from state to state, program participants should list the name of the units (e.g., Office of Adult Health or Division of Nutrition), and describe how they partner with the state CVH Program. They should also provide information on how the state CVH program coordinates and works with other CDC-funded programs.

B. **Formal Partnerships:** Partnerships involving a written or verbal agreement and involvement and commitment on a committee or work group necessary for the developing a state cardiovascular plan, a state CVH program, interventions, or activities specified in either.

C. **Informal Partnerships:** Partnerships involving occasional contacts and sharing of information for developing a state cardiovascular plan, a state CVH Program, or interventions or activities specified in either.

D. Commitment of Partners: CDC expects that partners will be involved in state CVH programs at different times and in different ways. Partners will contribute a variety of resources and skills during the development, implementation, evaluation, and modification of the state CVH plan.

Primary prevention: Preventing CVD risk factors and first cardiovascular disease events.

Policy:
A. Public Policy: A formal statement of standards by a public official, or legislative body, or by the general election of the public.
B. Organizational Policy: A formal rule and/or regulation that governs behavior and practice within an organization or in a particular setting.

Population-based strategies: Interventions that focus on an identified population (e.g., women age 35-65) or community (e.g., residents of Madison County) rather than on individual behavior change. Strategies should include policy and environmental approaches to improving cardiovascular health and the public education necessary to create a consensus for such approaches.

Priority Populations: Population groups that have higher documented rates of cardiovascular diseases and related risk factors, less access to services, or lower socioeconomic status than the general population.

Secondary Prevention: Activities designed to prevent further cardiovascular disease and to promote cardiovascular health, among people with established CVD. These activities include efforts to change polices and environmental factors related to CVH.

Settings: The locations or channels where interventions are implemented. The CVH State Program targets worksites, schools, health care facilities, and community settings such as churches and grocery stores.

Special State Surveys: Special one-time surveys to assess a state's cardiovascular disease burden or community awareness about CVD or to guide the formation of interventions and program planning.

Support: For purposes of the CVH State Program evaluation, "support" is defined as information sharing, and the dedication of resources or in-kind contribution to the state CVH program in that state.

Technical Assistance: The giving of advice or consultation on specific issues relating to CVH and the CVH State Program activity.

Training: The transfer of information in a structured situation that increases the skill level of public health professionals and CVH partners and enhances the ability of the CVH State Program to achieve its goals.

Appendix B
Overview Logic Model

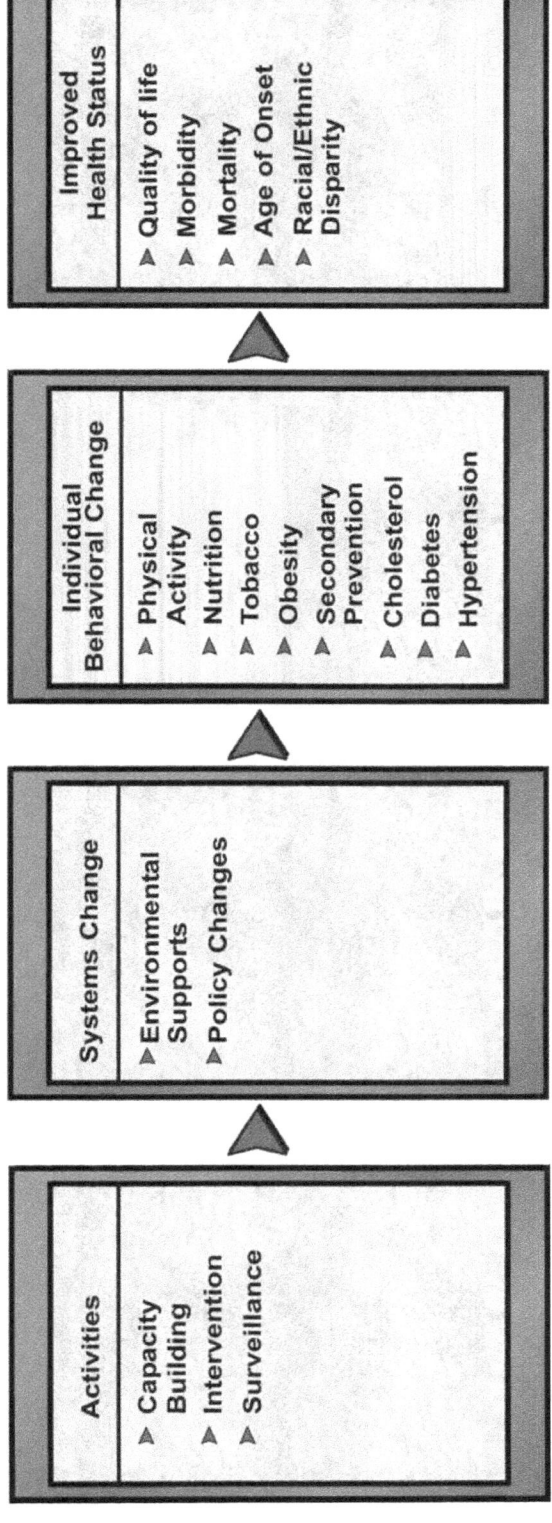

Activities
- Capacity Building
- Intervention
- Surveillance

Systems Change
- Environmental Supports
- Policy Changes

Individual Behavioral Change
- Physical Activity
- Nutrition
- Tobacco
- Obesity
- Secondary Prevention
- Cholesterol
- Diabetes
- Hypertension

Improved Health Status
- Quality of life
- Morbidity
- Mortality
- Age of Onset
- Racial/Ethnic Disparity

1

Appendix C
Expanded Logic Model

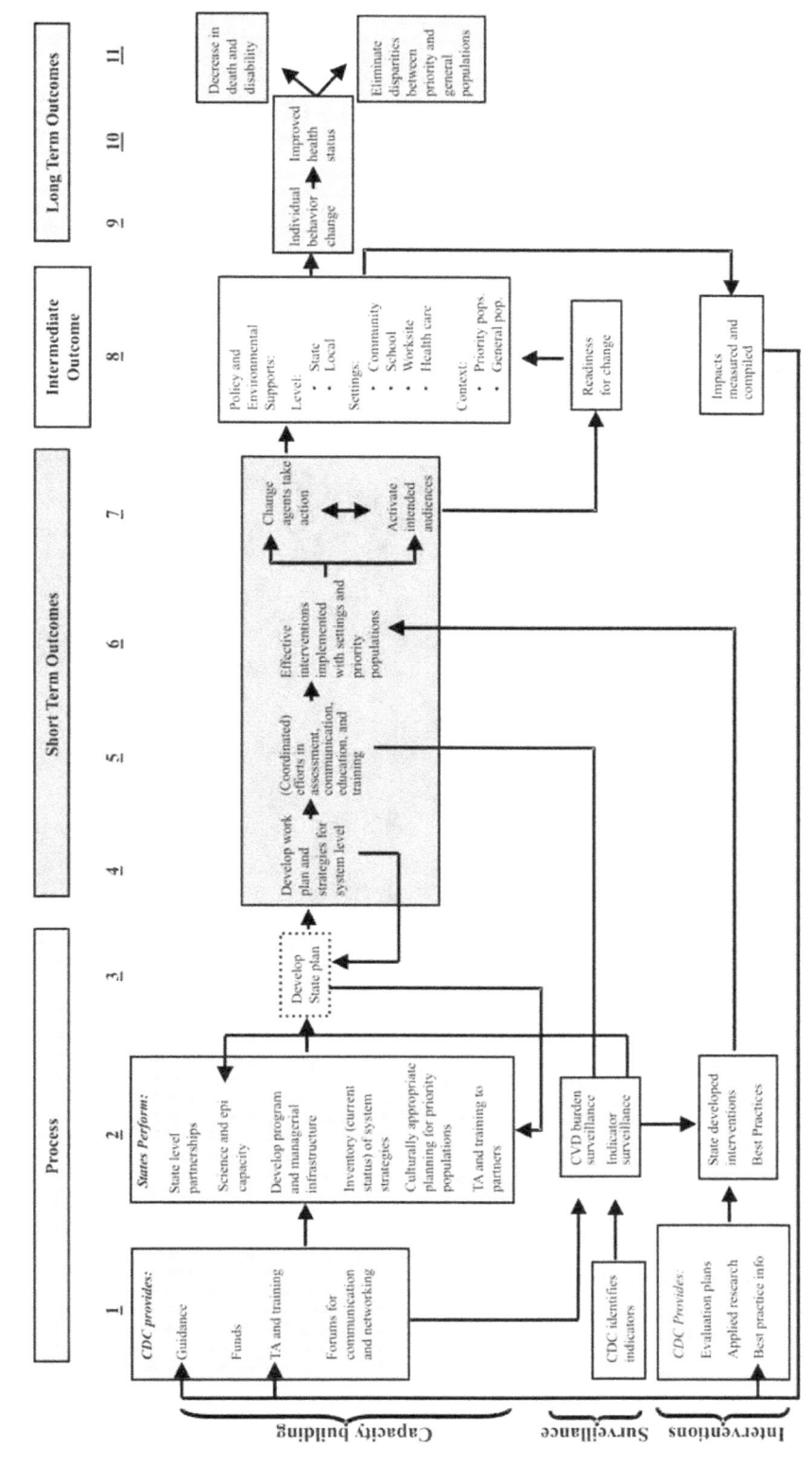

Appendix D
Logic Model Narrative

The first logic model is an overview model that presents, in broad outline, key program and the sequence of intended effects. The second model provides more detail on activities and is intended to depict the relationship among and between the activities and the sequence of intended effects.

- Logic models are intended to represent the *ideal*. That is, they depict intended activities and the effects of those activities *if things go as planned*. Of course, reality may be much different, especially in the early years of the program.

- These logic models depict the activities and effects intended by *CDC's funding* for these CVH programs; however, CDC may be only one of several funding sources, and the logic model for the state's overall CVH efforts may be more elaborate than these models.

<u>Overview Logic Model</u>

- CDC provides or enables the provision of guidance, funds, technical assistance and training, and opportunities for communication and networking among the sites.

- These inputs provided by CDC and others are the platform for state activities in three areas:

  - **Capacity building**
  - **Surveillance**
  - **Interventions**

- Over time, these activities result in system-level changes including changes in CVH-related policies and legislation and environmental conditions. These changes may happen directly as a result of the activities, or, more commonly, because these activities influence key change agents who can control CVH-related policy and environmental conditions.

- Changes at the system level frame/encourage/channel individual behavioral change, including the adoption of primary, and secondary, prevention practices related to CVH.

- ▸ This is the engine that affects long-term outcomes such a CVD stage at detection, patients' age at onset of CVD morbidity and mortality rates, and the elimination of CVH disparities between general and racial/ethnic populations.

Expanded Logic Model

This model provides more detail on the three types of state activities, the relationships among the activities, and relation of activities and the sequence of outcomes.

Capacity Building

- **CDC provides** guidance, funding, technical assistance, training, and opportunities for states to network with each other.

- This allows states to build program and managerial infrastructure; form partnerships at the state level; build the scientific, epidemiologic, and evaluation capacity they need to identify and monitor progress on key CVH issues; conduct ongoing inventories and assessments of system supports; and develop plans for addressing CVH in priority populations, as well as permitting states to train on these same issues with their partners.

- These capacity-building activities serve as a "platform" for developing a state plan, or, in the absence of a state plan, a CVH work plan and system-level strategies that address key settings and priority groups. However, in the early years of a program, the work plan may mostly involve developing a state plan and/or building up capacity, rather than the way it is depicted in the model with the platform and state plan informing the work plan.

- Work plans and strategies may include **coordinated efforts in communication, education, and training**. These affect development , **implementation, and effectiveness** in various settings.

- These interventions have the following as their intent: (1) changing knowledge, attitudes, and behaviors of system **change agents** so that change agents will take action, and (2) activating key **target audiences** so that they will be both receptive and ready to take advantage of policy and environmental change, as well as help advocate with change agents. There is also likely to be interaction between the change agents and intended audiences which will influence the change agents to take action.

- Action taken by change agents results in **policy and environmental supports** at the state and local levels and in various settings and contexts.

- Activation of intended audiences also results in a **readiness for change** in the community and individuals which influences ability to modify policy and environmental supports.

- Impacts of efforts on system change are measured, compiled, and fed back into (1) future State work plans, and (2) CDC-compiled "models that work" and guidance to all CVH States.

- These system changes provide the environment which supports **individual behavior change** over time, including adopting primary prevention practices related to CVH.

- Individual behavior change leads to **improvements in long-term health status**, with an ultimate decrease in death and disability and eliminating CVD disparities between general and priority populations.

Surveillance
- States undertake two classes of surveillance: (1) **surveillance of CVD burden**, and (2) **surveillance of progress** on policy and environmental supports.

- **CDC provides surveillance guidance** to States for both burden and policy/environmental surveillance using a set of selected system-level indicators. These indicators inform, but do not necessarily exhaust, the policy and environmental support indicators a State may chose to include in its surveillance (e.g., monitoring secondary prevention strategies).

- States **implement surveillance** activities.

- Surveillance results provide CVH information which is used in **program planning** to refine and improve programs and program implementation, as well as to inform development and improvement of **interventions**.

- Surveillance system measures State progress on CVH status, and *in the long term*, <u>may</u> be able to detect the impact of interventions.

Interventions

- CDC provides evaluation guidance/plans, applied research, and "models that work" (best practices) information for measuring processes and impacts.

- Informed by the work plan, strategies, and CDC guidance, **States and their partners develop and undertake interventions** in priority settings and with priority groups.

- These interventions capitalize on efforts to sensitize/activate change agents and target audiences.

- **Interventions strive to change systems** at the state, local, and setting level.

- **Impacts of interventions** on system change are measured, compiled, and fed back into (1) future State work plans, and (2) CDC-compiled "models that work" and guidance to all CVH States.

- These system changes provide the environment which supports **individual behavior change** over time including adoption of primary prevention practices related to CVH.

- Individual behavior change leads to **improvements in long-term health status**, with an ultimate decrease in death and disability, and eliminating CVD disparities between general and priority populations.